HEALING MENTAL ILLNESS

Lessons Learned in the Trenches

Joshua Alexander

Copyright © 2019 Joshua Alexander.

All rights reserved. No part of this book may be used or reproduced by any means, graphic, electronic, or mechanical, including photocopying, recording, taping or by any information storage retrieval system without the written permission of the author except in the case of brief quotations embodied in critical articles and reviews.

Disclaimer: This book is an account of personal experiences, and the thoughts or opinions expressed herein are not to be taken as a substitute for professional advice. Please consult with a licensed health care practitioner as needed.

The author of this book does not dispense medical advice or prescribe the use of any technique as a form of treatment for physical, emotional, or medical problems without the advice of a physician, either directly or indirectly. The intent of the author is only to offer information of a general nature to help you in your quest for emotional and spiritual well-being. In the event you use any of the information in this book for yourself, which is your constitutional right, the author and the publisher assume no responsibility for your actions.

TO every person living today who has been diagnosed with mental illness or is struggling with symptoms, my heart goes out to you. Know that you are not alone, and that there is a path forward.

AND TO all of the people who have been diagnosed with mental illness over the centuries, including my grandmother, who have been misunderstood, mistreated, drugged, locked away in asylums and sanitariums, and subjected to barbaric treatments, I am so sorry. Society was not ready for the level of healing that you needed, but we are now. Your sacrifices will not be forgotten.

TABLE OF CONTENTS

PART I – HEALING MENTAL ILLNESS

    CHAPTER 1: INTRODUCTION

    CHAPTER 2: STAGES TO HEALING

- Medication
- Alternative Treatments
- Homeopathy

    CHAPTER 3: HEALING THE ROOT CAUSE

PART II – PRINCIPLES FOR MENTAL HEALTH

    CHAPTER 4: SPIRITUALITY

- Coping with Trauma and PTSD
- Powerlessness, Surrender & Grace
- Loving God, Peace & Joy

    CHAPTER 5: PRACTICES

- Address the Physical Root Cause
- Maintain Daily Routines
- Be True to Yourself

- Seek the Truth
- Adapt
- Build a Foundation with Slow Growth
- Have Personal Responsibility
- Follow Universal Principles

PART III – HEALING AFTER HEALING

    CHAPTER 6: HEALING IN BODY

    CHAPTER 7: FINDING JESUS

    CHAPTER 8: THE SIMPLE LIFE

    CHAPTER 9: CONCLUSION

PART I -
HEALING MENTAL ILLNESS

CHAPTER 1: INTRODUCTION

When I finished writing *Healing Schizoaffective*, I had been medication free for over two and a half years. After a decade long battle with mental illness, I felt that I had beat it. I was no longer dependent on medication, and to me, that meant I was free from the illness. Everyone faces challenges and struggles in life, but they make do, they get by. They adapt. To me, not being dependent on medication, i.e. being able to function without medication, meant that I no longer had schizoaffective disorder, that I was healed.

If you read my first book, then you will know that I used medication as a tool when I needed it. I absolutely respect everyone's unique journey and free-will choices that they have to make with the resources that they have. If you are taking medication and it is helping, then I salute you. God bless you. I am only writing this book to share the insights and tools that I have learned on my own extremely painful and challenging journey, to try to save people from some of the suffering that I went through.

If you can glean some wisdom from my experience with mental illness, then it might help to inform your own journey, or that of your loved one, or your patients, to save some time and pain. If you read this book as just that, my own take on my own journey, then you can read it with an open mind and an open heart, and just take what applies to you or what works for you, and leave the rest.

I have a friend who experiences depression and anxiety and takes medication for it, and he works a high-stress job as a corporate attorney. He has a family, and takes vacations, and lives a full life. He may choose to be on medication for life. However, there are other people, like myself, whom that wouldn't work for. I just want you to have choices. I want you to have the freedom to heal in a way that offers you the opportunity to live a blessed and meaningful life.

I know how challenging mental illness can be. I've been locked up against my will. I've been told I would have to lower my expectations for my life. I've had to choose between taking oral medication against my will or being held down and given an injection. I've had to choose between living in a homeless shelter or a group home for the mentally ill.

I've felt such powerlessness and despair that I no longer wanted to live. I've had chronic stress levels so high, for so long, that it felt like my nerves were frying. I've felt broken in body, mind, heart, and soul. There have been times when I've faced challenges so great, that I laughed out loud because I literally couldn't believe how hard my life was. I've cried until there was nothing left. I've screamed until there was nothing left. There were times that I've felt like I sweat tears.

My point in telling you all this is that I know how hard it is. I've been there. It's been nearly sixteen years since my diagnosis, and over six years that I have been medication-free. I've learned some things along the way. I also know how we can move forward, how mental illness can be overcome. I know that healing is possible, and I want you to know it too!

May God bless you on your journey, always. Have faith, have hope, just do the best you can, little by little, day by day, and know that you will move forward eventually. You are not alone, you matter, and your struggles matter. They are helping to heal a broken world.

CHAPTER 2: STAGES TO HEALING

There were many stages to my illness, and steps to my journey. There was a period of time when I didn't know that I was sick, and another where I accepted that I had an illness. My recovery process was very long, and I had to use many different tools along the way. Your journey might look different than mine. You may be able to skip over some of the steps that I went through, or they may not be in the same order. The point is to keep learning, and as your understanding evolves, and your view of the cycles of the illness becomes larger, and you learn new tools that are effective, the illness becomes smaller.
Over time, you can make progress. Then, when you find yourself back in a situation that looks familiar, or you feel like you're repeating the same mistakes, you will learn a little more each time, or you will be better equipped to handle it. Eventually, the cycles back get smaller, the steps forward get longer, and you keep gaining ground until you are out of the woods and the illness is far enough behind you.

Medication

Taking medication was one stage of my recovery process. It served a purpose, and it was there when I had no other tools to use. It helped me to maintain some stability so that I could start piecing together my broken life. I was able to work a simple job and function for periods of time. However, I felt absolutely terrible. I felt dead inside, like I could never truly fulfill my potential. I felt like my life would be a pale settlement for what it could actually be. I couldn't bear not being myself.

Alternative Treatments

I had tried many other things to heal. I tried diet and exercise, self-help books, socialization, and spiritual practices such as meditation. I ate the healthiest foods that I could, tried to live as clean a life as possible, and I still couldn't break free. I also tried alternative treatments. My parents paid two thousand dollars at a clinic for me to have a PET-scan of my brain, so that they could recommend the "right" medication. I ended up feeling worse on what they recommended.

I worked with different therapists, psychologists, and psychiatrists, trying to help me to move forward. While it was helpful to talk to someone and it provided temporary relief, it didn't produce lasting change for me.

I visited an alternative residential treatment center in Arizona that was using a combination of techniques including orthomolecular medicine. I met with the founder in hopes of finding an answer, but I was not convinced enough to try it and didn't have the many thousands of dollars that it would have cost to do the program.

Homeopathy

It wasn't until I found homeopathy that I experienced a marked improvement and lasting change in my life. Homeopathy enabled me to function in my life without medication. This meant that I would no longer have to experience the negative side effects of the pills, such as feeling emotionally numbed, lethargic, mentally dull, and just feeling a general sense of being unfulfilled. It was a game-changer!

Without having to be on medication, but no longer having to face inpatient hospitalizations, I could apply my full faculties and effort into improving my life. This new hope and the excitement at having the chance to actually live my life the way that I wanted to, just fueled my drive. (If you'd like to learn more about how homeopathy helped in my recovery, see *Healing Schizoaffective*.)

When *Healing Schizoaffective* was published in May of 2016 I was living my life. I had been married, bought a home, and was working a full-time, salaried position. I felt that I was out of the woods with the illness, and for the most part I was. However, I didn't realize the trauma that I was carrying and the continued healing that would have to take place.

These past three and a half years have been incredibly challenging and I've learned so much and experienced healing more deeply than I knew I needed. I now feel that I've gotten all of the claws of the illness out of me, and that I've healed the root cause, so that I no longer have the illness. I am fully healed.

The first test came the same month that my book was released when there was a death in my family. When I was younger, I didn't realize the impact this could have. This, combined with financial pressures and other life stressors, was too much for me. I was having a hard time handling my responsibilities and was starting to feel unstable. I was feeling a little too wired, and was starting to lose sleep.

Since my book had just been released, where I said I was healed, I didn't want to acknowledge that I was sick. In truth, I was starting to relapse. My wife and naturopathic doctor were trying to get me to go back on homeopathy, despite my resistance. Thankfully I listened, and the homeopathy pulled me out of it again. I was able to avoid being hospitalized or going back on medication, but it was a close call. This experience only served to prove to me again the effectiveness of homeopathy.

Part of the reason I think I was resistant to going back on homeopathy, aside from not wanting to admit that I was sick again, was that I had discovered what I thought, and still believe, is the root cause of the illness, and the information and tools to heal it. In homeopathy, they say that the remedy causes the body to go back into balance so that it can heal itself. This may be true with conditions that the body can heal on its own, given the right environment and/or supports. However, I didn't feel like this was the case with me.

The homeopathy was keeping me in balance relative to my external environment, but when things in my life shifted, the remedy or dosage would have to be changed. Maybe given enough time, if I could build enough supports and structure in my life, I would be able to live and thrive without the remedies. This just wasn't good enough for me. I wanted to heal the cause, so that I could be free, so that I wasn't dependent on medications, or remedies, or anything else for my "illness." I wanted to be truly and fully healed of it.

CHAPTER 3: HEALING THE ROOT CAUSE

The previous year, in early 2015, I discovered the Medical Medium. My wife introduced it to me (she has a habit of finding the things that save my life, as she was also the one who found homeopathy for me), and she had me listen to one of his radio show episodes. I could hear the truth, authenticity, and compassion in his voice, and I knew with all my being that it was the truth. I know the truth when I hear it. It was from the Medical Medium that I learned about toxic heavy metals.

Toxic heavy metals are something that most people don't think about too often. We don't see them, because they are microscopic or nanoscopic particles, and so "out of sight, out of mind." "What you don't know can't hurt you," as it is supposed to go. In reality, human beings on planet earth are being and have been exposed to large amounts of toxic heavy metals for a long time, including mercury, aluminum, lead, copper, cadmium, nickel, and arsenic.

According to the Medical Medium, our food is laden with toxic copper from pesticides, herbicides, and fungicides, our water has metals in them from copper pipes, we get metal from fluoride treatments (which is an aluminum byproduct), heavy metals are falling out of the sky from jet planes, we get mercury in us from early standard medical treatments, and even pharmaceuticals have toxic heavy metals in them (*Medical Medium Liver Rescue book, pages 278-279*).

The truth is that we get toxic heavy metals in us. The Medical Medium explains that they collect in the liver and the brain, and contribute to all manner of ills (*Medical Medium book, page 259*). Aside from intuitively knowing that it's the truth, I believe in the Medical Medium information because it works. If you go to the Medical Medium Instagram page, *@MedicalMedium*, there are hundreds of testimonials over the past few years from people who have healed all sorts of chronic illness by following the information, and I'm one of them.

When I started following the information and implementing the changes in my life in 2015, I knew that I had found the answer. I just didn't know how long of a process it would be. Now that I have been following the information for over four years, I have a little more perspective.

One of the main tools that he recommends for heavy metals in the body is the Medical Medium Heavy Metal Detox Smoothie (*Medical Medium Celery Juice book, pages 151-152*). It pulls the metals all the way out of the body, slowly and gently. The five ingredients bind onto the metals and pass them like a football until they are eliminated. I highly recommend reading the chapter in his first book, *Medical Medium*, called "Freeing the Brain and Body of Toxins." The five ingredients are: Barleygrass Juice Powder, Spirulina, Atlantic Dulse, Cilantro, and Wild Blueberries. You can find links to the products on *MedicalMedium.com* on the supplement directory tab.

(*Note: the Medical Medium doesn't sell supplements, doesn't have sponsors on his podcast, doesn't charge for online courses, and doesn't have ads on his YouTube channel. The only thing that he sells are the books to get the information out there so people can heal. One of the main tools that he recommends, drinking at least 16 oz of fresh, straight celery juice every morning on an empty stomach, does not make him money. Celery farmers don't even make a lot of money. The Medical Medium is one of the most selfless, humble, compassionate servants of the highest good that I have ever had the honor of hearing speak.*)

After about a year of drinking the Medical Medium Heavy Metal Detox Smoothie every day, I started to feel a mental clarity that was significant. This happened to coincide with the summer of 2016 when I was having my minor relapse. I guess when the metals are pulled out of the brain over time, they leave microscopic holes that then need to be filled in, as the brain adapts with new experiences.

I also believe that removing the root cause of my illness started to make me aware of the underlying trauma. I didn't realize how "damaged" I was from all of the horrifying experiences that I'd been through. I didn't realize how broken my heart was from all the hurt, and the losses, and the strained relationships.

Thankfully I had the homeopathy to help me weather the acute storm of that summer, but it would take the next few years to heal and work through all of the trauma, which I am still doing. Each year I feel marked improvements and my health gets better and better. I am still taking the Heavy Metal Detox Smoothie every day, as well as drinking celery juice, taking some of the recommended supplements, and implementing the other Medical Medium information, as I will continue to do for the rest of my life, so long as it is within my power.

I can't stress this enough, if you're dealing with depression, anxiety, bipolar, schizoaffective disorder, schizophrenia, or any other form of mental illness, the Medical Medium information has answers. It is the highest truth in health information, and it is the only source that I trust. All other information is contaminated by man-made theories, profit-driven agendas, mistakes born of ignorance, or other ulterior motives (not by the doctors but by the industries).

There's no way that I can convince you of this though. Ultimately, each of us must use our own discernment and search for the truth, take responsibility for our own life and our own health, and choose for ourselves. I pray that you choose wisely.

PART II -

PRINCIPLES FOR MENTAL HEALTH

CHAPTER 4: SPIRITUALITY

Coping with Trauma and PTSD

Over the next two and a half years, I continued to be tested and challenged beyond my capacities. By late 2016, still in a weakened state from my minor relapse that summer, I was feeling tremendous financial pressure in regards to our home. I didn't realize the amount of time, energy, and money required to maintain and upkeep a house. I kept getting hit with one thing after another. Our gravel driveway washed out with the rain, then we had a plumbing leak. Then a toilet lever would break, or a sink would get clogged, not to mention regular lawn mowing and snow plowing.

Also, each piece of equipment needs to be maintained, which requires more time, energy, and money to learn how to do. My rider mower broke down, so I paid to have it fixed. Then it still wasn't working properly so I had to hire a lawn-mowing service.

It was just one thing after another and each time another thing broke, it was like something cracked inside of me. My nervous system felt fried from decades of chronic stress beyond what I could bear, and I felt like I just couldn't handle anymore stress. It felt like I didn't have the wit or the strength to solve these problems as they arose, and it was tearing me apart inside.

When the stress levels crossed my tolerance threshold I would have outbursts of rage. I would scream and swear, or go into my garage and grab a broomstick and start smashing boxes of things. I would kick the side of my car. If this happened while I was driving I would punch my radio console. I broke it twice and had to go to a junkyard to get a replacement. After the third time I just left it broken, so I've been driving without a radio for over a year now.

It reminded me of scenes from a movie where a war veteran is back home and having uncontrollable outbursts of rage, that are disrupting his family. This was taking a terrible toll on my marriage, but no matter how hard I tried, or how many tools and techniques I implemented in my life to try to maintain stability, I couldn't stop it. My guilt and feelings of failure only added to my burden.

Powerlessness, Surrender & Grace

I had experienced this level of powerlessness during my illness, when I was unable to hold down a job or meet my required responsibilities for survival, but I had just attributed this to the illness. Now that I was functioning enough in my life to get by, and I couldn't blame the illness, it was very eye opening for me. I really got to the bare-bones of myself and was tested in a new way where I could have self-reflection.

I have always tried to be a good person, have integrity, be kind, obey the law, and be helpful to others. Getting to a point where despite my best effort and discipline I was unable to be who I wanted to be, taught me a lot. On the weekends when I was stressed and tired from work, and I just wanted to rest and recover, when problems would arise I would say things like "I can never get any reprieve." It seemed like nearly every time I wanted to relax there would be challenges in my way. My typical response was to throw my adult tantrums and blame society or God. I didn't understand why I couldn't get what I needed.

What happened was, the pain and suffering birthed me into a new place. My own powerlessness forced me to surrender. Rather than thinking "I never get reprieve," I started thinking things like "here we go again," or even, with rebelliousness, "let's do this, bring it on!" There were times when this took the form of not caring. My car would break down and rather than worrying about how I would pay for it or blaming God, I would think "do what you will to me, I don't care."

As my suffering became acceptance and surrender, I started to notice that things always seemed to work out. I started to experience a grace that I had never known before, and I started to trust in God. This allowed for me to be less concerned with "what's going to happen to me," and focus more on being of service, which is what I really wanted to be doing anyway. Little by little, the fear was being replaced with trust and I began developing a love relationship with God. I hadn't really understood before the concept of loving God, or how to do it, but I was beginning to learn.

Loving God, Peace & Joy

Through my daily prayers I was actually starting to feel gratitude. I knew that I was failing and falling short every day, and that all of my strength and intelligence wasn't enough, but I was still getting by with the grace of God. Even though I was still suffering and struggling, and facing challenges, I had a peace within that surpassed understanding.

My newfound experience of grace didn't mean that I could just sit back and relax as the blessings flowed to me. I was still giving all I had and doing my best to survive and thrive, but I knew now that there was a safety net. As long as I was doing my best and being honest with myself in my heart and mind, God wouldn't let me fall too far. This doesn't mean that I always understand my challenges or why God doesn't deliver me from them, but I am okay with it.

For example, in 2016 we decided to put our house on the market in part to help reduce the financial pressures and maintenance responsibilities that I was referring to earlier. It wasn't selling, and I didn't know if it was because God wanted us to keep the house or not, or if it even mattered. It's been three and a half years and the house still hasn't sold and I still don't know. However, I have let go of the outcome.

My financial situation hasn't improved, but I know that I have enough to get by. I know when I wake up each morning that I'll be able to get through the day, and if I just live one day at a time, I'm okay. I used to wonder why I couldn't get ahead, and now I've stopped trying to. I do the best that I can today and I trust that the infinitely-loving, infinitely-intelligent Creator of the universe is orchestrating all things for the highest good.

I know that God's in charge, and I take comfort from this. I have enough, and that's enough. This allows for an incredible freedom of being where I can actually enjoy the simple things. I love prepping food and my spice rack brings me more joy that I can explain. Any time that I get to spend in nature is such a blessing. I see people with wonder and awe at their own uniqueness and how they adapt to their own life and what excites them and what they are interested in.

I am appreciating life more deeply in a way that I didn't know was possible. I am beginning to experience joy amidst the struggle, which has been an incredibly painful process, but it is also more magnificent than I ever could have imagined.

This growth process is much slower and more painful than I thought it would be. It is teaching me patience on a whole new level. Things don't always happen the way we want, or when we want. I wanted my house to sell and it hasn't. I wanted to increase my income and it hasn't despite my best efforts. I love Tesla cars, but I don't know how I'll ever be able to get one. Maybe I won't be able to own one myself, but I'll be able to ride in them when the self-driving is perfected, and the cars are available as part of the Tesla Network for ride sharing.

Mental illness is great at providing people practice at experiencing losses. The aches from the losses turn into an experience of letting go, and allow for us to experience subtler, but greater blessings. It's not something that we can necessarily think our way to. Life experiences birth us into new understanding.

Our busy-mind hates this because it requires being humbled and having our ego broken-down, which is a very painful process that feels like dying. It requires a level of honesty with ourselves that is hard to do. It's not easy to admit when we are wrong. My first inclination when I accidentally cut someone off in traffic is to try to rationalize it or blame the other person. To truly look within and ask myself, "did I make a mistake," or "could I have done better," hurts. To really acknowledge to myself, "I made a mistake, how can I learn from this and do better next time?" initially feels like unraveling, but quickly becomes feelings of peace.

This honesty in our own heart and mind is repentance, and I think that is why God asks this of us, not for Him, but for us. It frees us so that we can experience greater love. God sees into our hearts and minds, and so we're not fooling anybody but ourselves.

CHAPTER 5: PRACTICES

Address the Root Physical Cause

Despite all of these spiritual revelations that I have been sharing, I still had to address the root physical cause of my illness. My spirituality was one of the most important factors in my recovery and healing, because it helped to give me hope, to keep my spirit alive, and to strengthen my perseverance so that I kept fighting and seeking an answer. However, it wasn't able to heal the illness.

When I was bedridden with depression for a month, I don't think reading about grace would have gotten me out of bed. When my anxiety was so high that I had to pace back and forth, my spiritual beliefs didn't lesson it. When I was experiencing acute psychosis, I actually had some religious delusions, so thinking about religion wasn't helping. We still have to deal with the physical reality of the world we live in.

If depression, anxiety, and bipolar disorder are caused by a virus feeding on heavy metals, other chemical toxins, and certain foods like eggs, dairy, and gluten, and excreting a neurotoxin that is disruptive to neurotransmitters and neurons (*Medical Medium Celery Juice book, pages 51-54*), then we have to clean it up. We have to knock down our viral load, build up our immune system, remove the foods that feed the virus, and clean the chemicals and heavy metals out of our body.

Anyone who has experienced mental illness knows that you can't just think your way out of it. No matter how much money someone offered me, I couldn't bench press 1,000 lbs tomorrow. Maybe in a crisis situation to save someone's life I could lift a car with an adrenaline rush, but even then there are physical limits.

If bipolar symptoms and psychosis is caused by toxic heavy metal deposits in the brain, so that the neuronal impulses can't flow properly, then we're not going to be able to fix it with will power. Psychotherapy won't heal it. We have to get the metals out! If we don't know what the true cause of our illness is, and how to heal it, then we don't really have the freedom to heal, and without our health we can't really be free to live life to our full potential.

I could write this whole book about the Medical Medium information, but the Medical Medium books do a much more effective job at explaining it. I believe that it is our God-given right to have the freedom to heal. It is your right to read the Medical Medium books and decide for yourself what to believe, so you at least have choices and know what your options are. Become your own health expert so that you're not dependent on other people and anemic sources for answers.

Maintain Daily Routines

Since our understanding of the truth evolves over time, I have found it essential to have a daily routine to build upon. It acts as the skeleton of my growth process and gives me a structural foundation upon which to grow. It allows for me to gauge my progress by acting as a measuring stick when my life or external environment changes. When something affects my daily routine, I know that it is affecting me.

For example, if I stay up too late watching T.V., and then I'm too tired to read the Bible before bed, I take note of that and reflect on how I want to make adjustments. I pick right back up with my routine in the morning, and the next time it's getting late and I'm trying to decide if I should watch just one more *Star Trek the Next Generation* episode, I have a choice. I know that if I choose to watch another episode, then the chance of me reading the Bible diminishes greatly.

How strong I feel in my morning yoga practice tells me a lot. I've noticed that when I eat certain foods I'll feel weak in my practice a couple of days later. When I eat too much chocolate I've noticed that my mood is low the next day and that I feel tired and lose motivated for my own growth.

My daily routine has been a source of stability for me that has been tremendously helpful in recovering from mental illness, healing, and growing as a person. Here are some of the things that I do, though I'm sure each person will adapt their own routine to their own unique circumstances.

Routines that I have Kept Daily for Years:

- Brush my teeth.

- Take a shower.

- Drink a glass of water with lemon upon waking.

- Practice 20 min of gentle-to-moderate yoga.

- Drink at least 16 oz of fresh, straight celery juice on an empty stomach.

- Have the Medical Medium Heavy Metal Detox Smoothie (*Barleygrass Juice Powder, Spirulina, Wild Blueberries, Cilantro, Atlantic Dulse*).

- Take some of the Medical Medium recommended supplements (*such as Liquid B12 with methylcobalamin & adenosylcobalamin, Ester-C, L-Lysine, Liquid Zinc Sulfate, Lemon Balm*).

- Eat one to two salads (usually with spinach).

- Eat at least two red apples.

- Read the Bible.

- Pray to God.

The things that I don't do provide just as much of a measuring stick as the things that I do regularly. For example, I don't eat eggs, dairy, or gluten. If I'm in a situation where I start considering having something with gluten in it, like if I'm out socializing with friends, then I know I'm going off course. I don't trust myself because I know I'll just rationalize my behavior as I get further and further from where I want to be.

My daily routine is what keeps me on track, not my will power, and not because I'm a good person. The habits make the man. In college I was able to bench press 250 lbs. It wasn't because I was just a strong person, but because I had been working out for eight years and regularly conditioning my muscles to be stronger. I've had to use my daily routine in a similar way to rebuild my life after the catastrophic collapses from my mental illness.

Another thing that I don't do is I try not to swear. The frequency and intensity of my swearing is a direct gauge on how I'm doing. When I start saying the s-word or dropping the f-bomb I notice it and know that my patience is starting to wear thin and that I'm swaying off course. I try to breathe and reel it in and take steps to get back on track before it advances into a full-blown meltdown.

The hard part in that situation is making the right choice. When I'm feeling like that, part of me doesn't want to stop. My pride doesn't want to let go of the anger, even though I know it would be for the best. My rebel heart wants to play the child, rather than choose to be more mature. I win some and I lose some, and either way I try to have compassion for myself. I know that I've been hurt deeply and been through a lot, and I know that God loves me unconditionally, forgives me, and has compassion on me, even when I don't feel worthy of it.

Be True to Yourself

In order to develop our own personal daily routine, we need to have foundational principles that we believe in. I read the Bible because I believe it to be the truth and the word of God. I follow the Medical Medium information for the same reason. There are many people in my life, family and friends, who don't share my beliefs. Thankfully, over my lifetime, I have learned to be true to myself.

Growing up, I was bullied and teased a lot by other kids. I was made fun of and isolated. It was hard to go through at the time, but it taught me to not care what other people think of me. This allows me to stick with something that I know to be true, even when I don't have outside validation for it. It has been tremendously helpful for me in getting through some of the difficult situations that I've been in.

For example, if we accept for a moment that serious mental illness is caused by high levels of toxic heavy metals in the brain, which I believe that it is, then the mainstream approach doesn't provide a solution. I was told in effect "we're not sure what's wrong with you, but we think you've got bad genes." The only solution offered is medication that may dull the symptoms, but which also contains heavy metals. It felt like I was being decommissioned, and was told that I would have to lower the expectations for my life.

It was like society said "sorry kid, you don't get the life that you were meant to live, you're just going to have to settle for less." Well I'm sorry, but that didn't work for me. "Society, you're going to have to do better." If I didn't have this quality of being relentlessly true to myself, even when no one else around me believes me, I don't know that I could have followed the path that I did.

There have been times when I held inside a kernel of truth and protected it like a precious gem without any shred of support from anyone around me. The truth is between me and God and I don't need another person to agree with me. I don't need any outside validation. I just don't. Maybe I get some of that quality from my mother, maybe it was forged in me as a youth by being picked on all the time, but either way it has served me well. God uses all things for good.

Seek the Truth

Along with my quality of being true to myself, I also have the quality of relentlessly seeking the truth. I am constantly re-evaluating what I hold to be true, testing it in real-world circumstances, and self-reflecting to question if I am being completely honest with myself. Otherwise, it would be quite easy to become a dogmatic, arrogant, know-it-all.

What I consider to be truth, I've vetted. I don't believe it because someone told me to, or because I heard it somewhere, but because I've searched and searched and tried and tried, and I can't find anything else that is more true. I can't find anything else that better applies in my life. I'm not seeking my truth, but universal truth, the truth that stands up in all circumstances.

The truth defends itself, and because I approach it this way, I don't have to defend it to anyone else. I have enough faith in the truth that I don't have to be afraid that someone's going to sway me from it. It seems like it's the people who are really insecure in what they believe that have to fight the hardest to get others to believe it. Because my ego's not in it, I don't have to do that. I know what's true inside, and I know that the truth will be the only thing standing at the end. The truth is more solid than I am. All I can do is try to align myself with it.

Adapt

Even though I believe in the existence of universal truth, absolute truth, or God's truth, whatever you want to call it, we still have to adapt it the best we can in our lives. For example, it may be universally true that eggs feed pathogens in the body, meaning it applies to every person, in every circumstance, all of the time. However, someone may have chickens and not have enough money to buy food, and have to choose between eating the chicken eggs or starving.

In that situation, the relative truth, or the highest good given the circumstances, may be to eat the chicken eggs. That doesn't mean it won't feed pathogens, but that person may have to find other ways to stay healthy. Maybe they can grow some lemon balm, which is antiviral, and make tea with the leaves. We all have to adapt to our life circumstances, resources, and understanding of the truth. We have to do the best we can with what we have, and find a way to survive.

I have a hard time affording all of the supplements that I need to feel healthy. I am at a point where I feel "at capacity" every day. I give all I have to give every day, and I'm maxed out. That means if I try to exert more energy I might need more calories, or more rest time. I am constantly trying to improve efficiencies and reduce cost, and be the most effective that I can be in my personal life. Sometimes I pretend that I'm running my life like Elon Musk runs one of his companies.

Build a Foundation with Slow Growth

I adapt the best I can, but I still don't feel I have everything that I need. Any time I try to make a "push" for something, I know that I'm going to experience the backlash in some way. I've found that making small adjustments to the daily grind and my daily routine is the best way to move forward. It's a slower process, but builds a foundation that lasts.

If I want to get from point A to point B, I have to start where I am and build from there, and move in the right direction, rather than trying to make a leap. Maybe other people are able to do that, but because of the level of instability I've experienced in my life, I much prefer slow growth with a stronger foundation to fast growth with less stability.

Plus, I like the slow burn. When I go for a jog I much prefer to stay relaxed with steady, rhythmic breathing, and feel the dull ache in my legs, to the high intensity pain and shortness of breath that comes with a sprint. I actually like how the dull ache feels. It makes me feel alive.

Have Personal Responsibility

We must be true to ourselves, and in order to do that we have to take complete responsibility for ourselves. We can't be true to ourselves if we are allowing ourselves to be dictated by the people and circumstances around us. I just got to a point where I was so fed up with being negatively affected by my surroundings.

I get a whiff of someone's cigarette and I feel like it's literally displacing the life right out of me. Someone at work is not following the proper work flow and it's creating chaos for me. I'm jogging in the morning and a bunch of horse flies are dive-bombing my face. I just got so tired of being a victim all the time and blaming everything else for my own problems, that I decided I was done. I don't care what this world throws at me, I am the only one responsible for my own life. If I'm struggling then I'll take steps to get stronger, I'll take steps to live cleaner and be more disciplined.

Every time I feel hurt by the outside world it just motivates me to double down on my own health regimen. It's just a reminder to me. It actually helps to keep me on the path. It's practice. That doesn't mean that I still don't get upset when I smell a cigarette. I say "God help them," and then I up my game. I take some extra Vitamin C, or eat a little more fruit, or spend some time in nature getting fresh air.

Every time something negatively affects me, I look to myself and ask "what can I do?". "How can I be stronger, better, more loving?". "How can I have more of a positive impact?". All this does is empower me, and it's a much more effective approach than just being a victim and placing outside blame.

The more I take personal responsibility for my own life and my own health, the better I feel. Every day that I stick with something on my daily routine makes me feel more in control of my own life. I think we all want to be free on some level, at least free to be ourselves, and taking personal responsibility is an essential step towards our own freedom.

Follow Universal Principles

If I didn't have these qualities, of being relentlessly true to myself, and of taking 100% personal responsibility, I think it would have been very difficult for me to stay on the narrow path. You wouldn't believe the number of people who have tried to sway me, whether intentionally or unintentionally, from what I know is right and true.

Since I work for a health food company, health is a hot topic. I've told people that I follow the Medical Medium information, and that it healed me from a ten-year "incurable" chronic illness. I've told them some of the basic principles and tools. Some of my co-workers are open to it and have even started juicing celery. Others didn't want to hear about it.

One of my old co-workers was into macrobiotics, which talks about "expanding" and "contracting" foods, and incorporates fermented foods into the diet. I told him that I don't eat fermented foods because they pickle the liver over time, according to the Medical Medium information (*Medical Medium Liver Rescue book, pages 239-240*). He continued to offer me fermented products in spite of knowing this. In our conversations in the break room, he would also mention how he eats more grains and meats, as if to allude that I should too (as he sat there eating his hard-boiled eggs).

I couldn't help but get the feeling that he was trying to get me to change my diet not for my own benefit, but for his. He thought I was "out of balance" because he felt uncomfortable around me, so he was trying to influence me. It reminded me of when an alcoholic gets sober and all his friends want him to keep drinking. He didn't know my health history, the myriad of factors I was dealing with in my life, the decades of experience I have studying holistic health (including macrobiotics), or how I felt inside, but for some reason he thought he knew what was best for me.

Other co-workers of mine seem to practice energy balancing as well. If they feel high they eat something to make them feel low, or if they feel low they consume something to feel high. The problem is, this is all relative to the people around them. They have no idea what customers are going to come in through the door, or what new hires are going to start work, etc. There are an infinite number of factors in the universe and we can't control them or predict them. What they end up doing is just whatever feels good in the moment, being tossed around like a bottle at sea.

A much more sound approach is to base our decisions on true principles, and to follow the guidance of the Holy Spirit (or our Divine guidance). Living based on tried and true principles, or universal principles, means that we have a North Star, or something against which to measure ourselves. Rather than basing our decisions on relative truths that are constantly shifting with the tides, we base them on universal truths that are steadfast and true, and will be the same tomorrow, and the next day, and the next day. When our limited understanding falls short of discerning the truth in a situation, we can rely upon our Divine guidance, or the Holy Spirit, to lead our way. That guidance never fails us, even if we can't understand the whole picture in the moment.

Even my fellow Christians seem to be following an "energy balancing" approach when it comes to eating. It seems like their strategy is to just eat whatever anyone around them is eating, thus "staying in balance" with the people around them. Seeing as society is getting sicker and sicker, younger and younger, rates of chronic illness are increasing, and the life expectancy is starting to decline, I don't think this is such a great strategy. Getting sick with the people around us is not going to help anybody.

In the Old Testament God says he would drop a plumb line into the world (*Amos 7:8*), against which we would be measured. In the same way that we are asked to forge ahead with spiritual principles, by Jesus' example, I think we should forge ahead with health principles. The healthier we are the more good we can do in this world. Jesus said what comes out of our mouth defiles us but what goes into it doesn't (*Matthew 15:11*). Does that mean I can just eat chocolate cake all day every day?

It seems like some Christians think food doesn't matter. I agree that our spirituallly is more important, but we still have to address the physical. We have to make sure we meet our physical needs for survival, like shelter, food, water, and clean air. We need to make sure we're getting enough calories, and enough nutrients. Are you telling me that no Christian has ever went on a diet program, or tried eating healthier? Our physical health is important no matter how spiritual we are, and we need to be sure we're basing it on sound, natural principles, not man-made, profit-driven ones.

As someone who grew up on organic health food, I am in awe when I go to church functions and see dishes of white flour with white sugar, cheese, coffee, and basically the worst of what the standard American diet has to offer. I've often thought that when Christians discover healthy eating (real health from the fruits, vegetables, leafy greens, and herbs that God created, not the packaged products and health food trends propagated by advertising), the forces of darkness in this world won't stand a chance.

As is evident every Sunday morning when my fellow church goers ask for prayers for themselves or their sick loved ones, Christians are not immune to chronic illness. The same people who serve money that we stand against are duping us with our food. The devil doesn't only manipulate us through the obvious vices, but through unseen ways like when a leading chemical company ghost-writes some "science" to keep us from knowing that what we're being exposed to is harmful. We have to be shrewder when it comes to our health and that of our loved ones, and we have to align ourselves with universal principles of health, not ones that were manufactured by some company to get us on board with their trendy products or diet programs.

PART III -

HEALING AFTER HEALING

CHAPTER 6: HEALING IN BODY

Each year that I follow the Medical Medium information I feel better and better. I think it takes time to get the toxins and heavy metals out, knock down the viral loads and pathogens, and to re-mineralize and re-hydrate the body. People don't realize how malnourished they are because of the way our food system has been manipulated. We gorge on empty calories full of MSG, under the guise of "natural flavors" to keep us eating, but we are starving for true nutrients.

I think it took me a long time to rebuild my glucose reserves, or glycogen storage. I had to "fill up" over a number of years with mineral salts from celery juice and leafy greens, and glucose from fruits and starchy vegetables, before I started to feel real good, full, strong, and healed in body.

According to the Medical Medium, nutrients don't enter our cells without glucose and when there is too much fat in the blood it blocks the sugar from entering the cells (*Medical Medium Liver Rescue book, page* 107). The high protein high fat, low carb (profit-driven) trends of the past few decades have also contributed, I believe, to people's malnourishment.

We keep stuffing in the protein and fat which gives the illusion of us feeling strong and full, but any glucose and nutrient absorption into the cells is diminished, and the high fat in our blood also lowers our oxygen levels, which helps pathogens to thrive. (*See the Medical Medium Liver Rescue book, pages 247-257 for more information.*) We're starving our brain of glucose and oxygen, our brains are shrinking, and people wonder why the country seems like its gone mad.

Around the time I started to get sick in 2002, I had gone on a vegan diet. I didn't know what I was doing and I was just eating oatmeal every morning for breakfast and rice and beans for lunch and dinner. My mom had started one of the early high protein low carb diet trends, and my family was full-on with the protein obsession. "Where're you going to get your protein?" they would say over and over again like some kind of droids. I told them that everything we eat has protein in it, but it didn't matter.

The more she kept packing in the protein, the more intense and domineering I felt my mom become. Over the years I've watched her try a number of trendy high protein diets, as the names keep changing, all the way up to the current keto-craze. I've watched the cycles of her losing weight and putting it back on, binging on carbs and then blaming it on her will power (when it was really her body forcing her to get glucose to save her life).

I think my parents blame at least part of me getting sick on the vegan diet. I think there were a number of factors including my isolation, my experimentation with marijuana in college, and my stress and burnout from Cornell, but I now know that toxic heavy metals in my brain was the root cause. There was so much fear from my parents around the "protein" issue, as it has been ingrained in our society, that they had blinders on. My mom is still afraid of it and when I stop by her house she still regularly offers me meat. It's really sad.

When I got sick I had to go off the vegan diet at the time because I didn't have the knowledge or means to stick with it, and truth be told, I bought into the protein fear a little bit. There's no way I could have stayed vegan without the Medical Medium information. I needed the mineral salts from the celery juice and leafy greens and I had to get the heavy metals out with the Heavy Metal Detox Smoothie.

As a result of the trauma of that experience getting sick it has taken me years to get over my fear. When I started the Medical Medium information in 2015 I cut out red meat, but I was doing fish and turkey two to three times per week. After about a year I started just doing wild salmon a few times a week. Then, after about another year or so I was just doing some wild salmon and some sardines. I would try to lower it and go plant-based for a while but then I would get afraid and eat a can of salmon.

I think it was a combination of me needing to re-mineralize and fill up my glucose reserves, as I said before, as well as healing from my past trauma, but I was finally able to let go of the fear. I started to notice that the morning after eating some animal protein I would feel strong in my yoga practice, but the day after that I would feel so weak I could barely lift my limbs. When I would go a week or so just plant-based I would feel so strong and clear in my practice and throughout my day.

I started to notice these cycles and was aware of my fear around protein. I finally just decided to kick it and took the leap of faith, and I feel so much better now! I made an agreement with myself that I could eat as many fruits and vegetables as I want. If I'm hungry I allow myself to keep eating fruits and vegetables as much as I want. I would feel like I was eating too much, in part due to the stigma in our society about overeating, but then I realized that fruits and vegetables have much less calories than high-fat foods and animal products.

Plus, I don't drink alcohol or coffee, or indulge in many of the other things that people in our society do, so I'm going to eat as many fruits and vegetables as I want without feeling guilty. I love filling up on steamed potatoes and asparagus, squash, or other hearty plant-based meals in the evenings. I usually do raw fruits and vegetables for breakfast, lunch, and throughout the day.

It has taken me years of trying to be healthy to find a balance that works for me, and I was only able to do it with the Medical Medium information. Knowledge is power when it is based in truth. I have been studying the Medical Medium books and podcast episodes for over four years, and implementing the information through my own daily practice, which is longer than some people spend getting their degree or certification. In today's world of misinformation, we must truly become our own health experts.

CHAPTER 7: FINDING JESUS

In addition to healing my damaged body, I had to heal my emotional wounds and psychological trauma from all that I'd been through. It would have been nice if I had unlimited resources and could have taken a year off and laid on a beach somewhere and just worked on my healing. However, maybe that wouldn't have taught me what I needed to learn. Unfortunately, I didn't have a surplus of resources and my lessons continued to take the form of me being broken down.

Both 2017 and 2018 continued to bring stressors and life challenges. My powerlessness just kept getting more and more evident as I continued to fail to meet what was being asked of me. When I was young, I felt like I had unlimited internal resources, and when challenges arose I could just push a little harder. Now, when I feel at capacity everyday and I'm already giving all I've got, when challenges arise I have nothing more that I can give. I try to get a little ahead so that I can save for the inevitable "rainy day" but even that proves to be a struggle and I end up just treading water. Rather than trying to get ahead I try to just keep up with and hold onto what I already have. The only path available seems to be sacrifice.

When you combine this experience with the hurt that I have inside from all the losses I have already endured, and feeling unsupported in the ways that I needed by society and my family, my trauma started to become quite evident. It was a form of a personal reckoning. It was like my whole life had caught up with me, and I had to deal with it or die. There were times when I wanted to just lay down and die, but I couldn't leave my wife alone. She needed me. That wasn't an option no matter how much pain I was in or how tormented I was. I had to push on. I had to find a way.

While I had been spiritual since my college years, and had studied many eastern texts and traditions, for a few years at this point I thought Jesus was probably the greatest spiritual teacher. I had read the first couple books of the New Testament, and I could tell by the stories of what he did and said that his path of love was the best. I would sometimes go into a fit and curse someone for cutting me off in traffic, and yet he was beaten near death without crying out, and then nailed to a cross to die, and he prayed for his persecutors.

When religious leaders of the time were going to stone a woman for committing adultery, he drew a line in the sand and said "he who has not sinned cast the first stone" (*John 8:4-7*). He taught "turn the other cheek" and "judge not lest ye be judged." When asked if he should pay the head tax to Caesar he replied by asking whose face was on the coin. When the person said "Caesar's", Jesus said "give unto Caesar what is Caesar's and to God what is God's" (*Matthew 22:17-21*). Wow! As someone who has a healthy distaste for the money system this was so cool to me.

Jesus was like a real-life rebel superhero. So, I loved Jesus and I thought His message was to love others, and I tried to be like him. I tried to follow his teachings and his example.

By 2017 when I was having my personal reckoning, it became very clear how far from Jesus' example I was falling. No matter how hard I tried, no matter how disciplined I tried to be, I kept failing. Every day I failed. Moreover, in the larger context of my life I couldn't be what I needed to be. All my wit and all my strength wasn't enough.

I got to a point where I had to turn to God because I had nowhere else to turn. I experienced that I couldn't make it on my own, and started to realize the greater truth of Jesus. He really was the incarnation of God, conceived by the Holy Spirit. It was impossible for me not to fall short, or not to sin in some way. The sins of my whole life were catching up to me, and I could see that my reward was death, and there was no way I could out-think it or outsmart it or out-muscle it.

It became obvious to me, not as a dogmatic belief or thought, but as a lived experience, that Jesus really did save me. By dying on the cross and then rising again on the third day he conquered death. When I started to talk to him and understand His love for me and let him into my heart, I started to experience new life. Daily prayer became a means of survival for me.

Only by letting Jesus in and calling on God for help could I go on. It is by His power that I was saved, not my own. Jesus is the only thing that was able to free me from the chains of this world. I am a broken sinner who can't bear the weight of my own sins, and I am only here by the sacrifice of Jesus and the grace of God.

Once I had this experience of being saved, I started to experience a peace that was inexplicable. It was like God had wrapped me in a warm blanket. The problems and challenges in my life hadn't changed, but I was a new person and they had less hold on me. I am living for God in a whole new way, and I am at peace.

I know that the "balm in Gilead" is the only thing that could heal my broken heart and my fractured soul. It is the only thing that could heal the type of trauma that I'd been through. I accepted Jesus Christ as my personal Lord and Savior in the fall of 2017. I started to read the Bible every day and pray every day and talk to Jesus.

My life didn't change overnight, and I still struggle every day, but now I know that with God's help I can get through today. That's all I need. I know that I can get through today and that's enough. Over the past two years since then, I struggle less and less. I am learning to trust God and to surrender to His will. No matter what happens to me in this world, I know that I am with God, and so I am okay.

Everyday my wounds heal more and more, and I become a little more whole. I can't imagine ever living my life without knowing Jesus and I don't know how I got by before. It's like I finally stumbled upon the greatest mystery of the universe, that people have been shouting from the mountaintops for two thousand years. I was lost, but now I'm found. I actually understand what that means now.

CHAPTER 8: THE SIMPLE LIFE

All my life I was striving for something, to be somewhere that I wasn't. When I was thirteen I couldn't wait to be sixteen so I could get my driver's license. In high school I couldn't wait to get to college. My entire time in college I couldn't wait until it was over. Even in little ways, I was always trying to be someone that I wasn't, to add a new skill to my list, to build my resume, to get a promotion.

I've sometimes wondered where this incessant struggle for more started. It was like I was born into it, always trying to have more, be more, do more, get more. I realized that it is one of the great lies of our society, which I call "The Achievement Myth." Somehow it gets ingrained in us that if we just get the next thing, then we'll be happy. I think it's just another way that society gets us to keep consuming. If we have feelings of emptiness, loneliness, and lack of fulfillment, then we'll keep trying to fill it by paying for the next degree, or buying the next consumer item, or eating more chemical-laden empty calories. The problem is that it never works. It just leads to a dissatisfied life and disease.

I think on a deeper level we are just trying to feel loved. I have a cheap guitar that I bought years ago that I never really learned how to play. Every time I think that I should put some time and effort into learning how to play, it's so that I can play in front of other people and impress them with my skill. I don't actually enjoy playing enough to put in the effort just for the beauty of it. However, left to my own devices I'll prep food all day every day. I love chopping veggies and making different meals and using spices. I don't have to find extrinsic reasons to motivate myself to do it. I am internally driven to do it. The same goes for my daily routines. I stick to them because I love them and they make me feel fulfilled. It is who I am.

Human beings are naturally curious and creative and have a sense of wonder and desire to discover as children. Unfortunately for some reason, I would argue due to economic pressures, the mainstream system squeezes that out of us and teaches us to force ourselves to do things we don't want to do, in order to earn rewards. Our self-worth becomes conditional upon our performance, and we are taught that we have to keep achieving.

In a sense, we are trying to earn love. We want to be loved for how smart or successful we are, or how beautiful we are, or for our position, prestige, power, money, etc. Now that I know how loved I am by the Creator of the universe, it's like I am freed from all that. I no longer have to achieve to feel loved. I can just be me. It's like I've been set free and the world has lost its grip on me. A true musician will play music in front of a stadium of 10,000 people, a restaurant with ten, in a room by herself, or in a subway station, because she's not doing it for the fame or money, she's doing it because that's who she is.

Obviously we need to ensure that we meet our physical needs to survive in this world, but beyond that we can be who we want. We don't have to do anything to be worthy. Now, I would argue that doing something creative is better than sitting in front of the T.V. every day, but I believe that each of us already knows that inside and will feel dissatisfied in front of the T.V. for too long.

However, in order to be ourselves we have to get the claws of this society out of us, from the advertising and addictions and junk that is the status quo here. We have to unplug from social media, and cheap entertainment, and fast food, etc. in order to be free. It's very uncomfortable to do this because then we have to face the emptiness and underlying pain that we've been trying to cover up. We have to face our fears.

At this point in my life I've realized the immense value of the simple life. The less I listen to the advertising telling me to strive for material stuff or fame, wealth, beauty, etc., the happier I become. The less I participate in the consumer economy, the happier I am. I only buy things when they are absolutely essential, and I try to repair, borrow, or buy used whenever possible.

I don't like being a slave, whether it's to an addiction, to finances, or to material possessions. The more that I sacrifice these things, the more that I am free to pursue what really matters in life, the simple things. I have time to smell the roses, listen to a friend, observe the majestic beauty of nature, breathe in some fresh air, try some new spices when I'm preparing a meal, look after someone in need, look up at the stars, and find peace in my heart. It's ironic that life is a process of letting go, and the more we let go the more abundance we feel.

      Never underestimate the value of sacrifice, and I have to thank my illness for that. By forcing losses in my life my illness was actually helping to set me free. I am such a better person now than I was before, healthier, happier, kinder, more compassionate, gentler, wiser, and stronger. I actually like myself now and appreciate who I really am, flaws and all. I am starting to regain my lost child-like wonder. I am amazed at the deep joy and fulfillment that I get from the simple things and simple moments in my life now. Life is better than I ever dreamed it could be.

CHAPTER 9: CONCLUSION

If you take one thing away from this book, I hope it is the knowledge that healing from mental illness is possible! Not knowing was the hardest part for me. I don't want you to have to suffer like I did, so please, learn from what I've been through. Maybe it can save you some time so that you can heal more quickly than I did.

There are real answers for why you are suffering. My grandmother had schizophrenia and spent the remainder of her life drugged in a managed-care facility. I have been medication-free for over six years now, and I am functioning fine and am actually thriving. This is because the illness is not genetic, it's the result of viruses and toxic heavy metals that are passed down from generation to generation in utero, and that we continue to accumulate during our lifetimes. It's totally heal-able with the right information.

I didn't heal because I have anything special. I'm not great, Jesus is great. I'm no better than you are. The only thing that may make me different from another person is that I chose to have the courage and willingness to seek the truth and be true to myself, even in the face of objections from other people and society. As Jesus said, "seek the truth and the truth will set you free." I have no doubt that if you do this earnestly and honestly, while following your Divine guidance, you will find your way too.

I have outlined a path of healing from mental illness in this book, as well as in my first book *Healing Schizoaffective*, and in my blog and podcast on my website *HealingSchizoaffective.com*. Your path may not look exactly like mine, but at least now you have some tools and a framework to work with that I didn't have when I started.

I wish you the very best on your journey. Don't ever give up. Even when you give up, don't give up. You were made for this. Your life matters very much and you have a unique soul that contributes to the universe in a way that none other can. I'm in it with you, healing little by little, day by day. May God bless you always!

www.ingramcontent.com/pod-product-compliance
Lightning Source LLC
Chambersburg PA
CBHW070842220526
45466CB00002B/857